Mediterranean Diet Meal Prep and Recipes Cookbook for Beginners

2000 Days of Quick, Easy, Delicious, and Nutritious Mediterranean-Balanced Diet Recipes to Lose Weight and Live Healthier

Valerie R. Johnson

Copyright Page

All right reserved, no part of this publication may be republished in any form or by any means, including photocopy, scanning or otherwise without prior written permission to the copyright holder.

Copyright ©Valerie R. Johnson 2024.

☐

Table of Content

Introduction

In the hectic fabric of contemporary life, finding a balance between a nutritious diet and delectable food can be challenging. This cookbook "Mediterranean Diet Meal Prep and Recipes Cookbook for Beginners." Serves as your guide with over 2000 days of delicious, easy, and quick meals based on a Mediterranean balanced diet.

This recipe book is more than just a cookbook; it's a guide to a healthy lifestyle, a celebration of food, and a means of losing weight.

Regardless of reader experience level with the Mediterranean Diet, these pages are meant to satisfy their needs. We understand the challenges of modern life, particularly the desire for nutritious but easily prepared meals. This is an absolute treasure trove of recipes that will fulfill both your nutritional needs and your taste buds.

Each recipe is made to fit effortlessly into your daily schedule, offering a practical and long-lasting way to embrace a Mediterranean lifestyle.

Moreover; this cookbook is intended to meet your needs, understand your tastes, and help you achieve your objectives, whether they be weight loss, healthy living, or simply enjoying eating.

With so much going on in today's fast-paced world, it can be tough to find a pleasant and sustainable way to nourish your body. The Mediterranean diet offers both a solution and a change. This cookbook is an excellent resource for implementing a healthy Mediterranean cuisine into your daily routine. We realize that you are busy and need recipes that are simple and easy to include into your hectic schedule, so we created them with that in mind.

Visualize yourself enjoying every bite of a meal that both satisfies your taste buds and advances your nutritional goals. Flavor is a want that should not be ignored on the path to happiness. With our carefully curated recipe collection, you'll enter a world where vibrant flavors coexist with nutritious ingredients, elevating each meal to a celebration of both taste and nutrition.

We understand that you want to live a healthy, energetic life and have a lasting connection with food. The Mediterranean diet, which is built on centuries of culinary wisdom, is more than just a diet; it is a way of life that may help you achieve your health and wellness objectives. This cookbook will guide you through this traditional eating technique with joy and confidence.

We realize the hurdles you may experience as you want to improve yourself, since understanding the vast area of nutritional knowledge may be intimidating. This cookbook has all of the answers you need, whether you're unclear how to cook or frustrated with finding healthy yet quick meals. It transforms potential impediments into opportunities to advance your wellness goals.

As we turn the pages of this cookbook, consider yourself beginning on a new culinary and nutritional adventure. "Mediterranean Diet Meal Prep and Recipes Cookbook for Beginners" is more than just a cookbook; it's a travel companion that will help you accomplish personal development. Every meal in 2000 Days of Easy, Nutritious, and Quick Meals moves you closer to being a more energetic, healthier version of yourself.

Let us embark on a journey where every meal is a tasty and deliberate choice, and eating becomes a pleasurable, nutritious, and self-care experience when you follow the Mediterranean diet.

Understanding the Basics of Mediterranean Diet

What Is the Mediterranean Diet?

The term "Mediterranean diet" describes the customary eating habits of the countries bordering the Mediterranean Sea. There isn't a traditional Mediterranean diet. At least sixteen countries border the Mediterranean. Eating patterns vary across these nations and among their respective areas due to variances in culture, economics, geography, religion, ethnic background, and agricultural production. There are, nonetheless, some similarities.

A Mediterranean-style diet often consists of an abundance of fruits, vegetables, bread and other grains, potatoes, beans, nuts, and seeds; olive oil as the primary fat source; and small to moderate amounts of dairy, eggs, fish, and poultry.

Fish and poultry are more common in this diet than red meat. It also places a strong emphasis on minimally processed plant-based food. It's fine to drink small to moderate amounts of wine, usually with meals. Fruit is a common ingredient in desserts instead of sweets.

Origins and Philosophy: The Mediterranean Diet is based mostly on the culinary traditions of the countries that round the Mediterranean Sea. This is a long-term, balanced diet that places a strong emphasis on whole grains, lean meats, heart-healthy fats, and an abundance of fresh fruit. It's much more than just a meal plan; at its core, it's an idea that highlights the value of eating with loved ones and taking the time to savor every bite.

Key Components of the Diet: The Mediterranean diet has a wide variety of nutrient-dense foods that work well together to promote health. Olive oil is a staple of the diet and is well recognized for its heart-healthy monounsaturated fats. While fresh fruits and vegetables provide a range of vitamins, minerals, and antioxidants, whole grains provide a consistent source of energy. Lean proteins like fish and legumes add variety, while dairy and wine are served in moderation to complete the meal.

Heart Health and Beyond: An abundance of studies has shown the remarkable benefits of the Mediterranean Diet, particularly in terms of promoting heart health. The anti-inflammatory properties of olive oil and omega-3 fatty acids from fish work together to create a powerful combination that supports cardiovascular health.

This diet has been linked to heart health as well as longer life, improved cognitive function, and a decreased chance of chronic disorders.

Adopting a Mediterranean Lifestyle: The Mediterranean Diet is more than just a list of suggested foods; it's a way of life. It encourages mindful eating, savoring each meal, and appreciating the connection between food, culture, and community. This way of living entails taking pleasure in life's small pleasures, sharing meals with close friends and family, and getting regular exercise.

Getting started with the Mediterranean Diet: It's easy to make the move if you haven't tried the Mediterranean diet before. Starting with your meals, up your intake of fruits, vegetables, and whole grains. Enjoy lean meats, swap out high-fat dishes with heart-healthy olive oil, and recognize the simplicity of using seasonal, fresh ingredients. Eventually, you'll find a rhythm that works for you and helps you reach your health goals.

Adopting the core principles of the Mediterranean Diet embarks us on a journey that extends beyond just nourishment. It's a culinary adventure, a celebration of health, and an exhortation to adopt a lifestyle that looks after for the body and the spirit. As you celebrate the Mediterranean Diet, may you also enjoy the exhilaration of a vibrant existence and the classic allure of a table adorned with the bounty of the Mediterranean.

Scientific Principles of Mediterranean Diet

The Mediterranean diet is a well-balanced set of scientific principles that work together to support optimal health, rather than just tasty food. This dietary pattern transcends fads and offers a blueprint for well-being backed by solid scientific evidence. It is based on decades of research and is commended for its comprehensive approach.

- **Heart Health:** The Mediterranean Diet's cornerstone is olive oil, a powerful ally. The cardiovascular benefits of this liquid gold, which is high in antioxidants and monounsaturated fats, have been well studied. Eating a diet high in olive oil has been shown in scientific studies to help decrease heart disease risk factors, such as low LDL cholesterol and improved endothelial function.

- **Omega-3 Fatty Acids:** The diet's emphasis on fatty fish, which is strong in omega-3 fatty acids, is another scientific cornerstone. These essential fats have been connected to a number of health benefits, such as the mitigation of inflammation, preservation of cognitive function, and vital role in cardiovascular defense. The Mediterranean diet includes fish such as salmon, mackerel, and sardines, which is consistent with research demonstrating the importance of omega-3 fatty acids for overall health.

- **Antioxidant-Rich Diet:** The abundance of fruits, vegetables, nuts, and seeds in the Mediterranean Diet is all about optimizing the health benefits of antioxidants, not only about delicious flavors and eye-catching hues. These compounds have a major role in the prevention of chronic disorders and the improvement of cellular health by combating oxidative stress. Antioxidants are abundant in the diet, ranging from lycopene in tomatoes to polyphenols in red wine.

- **Balanced Macronutrients:** The Mediterranean Diet has the perfect macronutrient makeup. It combines lean proteins, healthy fats, and complex carbohydrates to create a nutrient-dense and sustainable meal. This balance promotes overall health by maintaining energy levels and satiety in addition to aiding in weight control.

- **Gut Health and Fiber:** A diet heavy in whole grains, lentils, and high-fiber foods promotes a healthy gut flora. Research has shown that gut health has a major influence on many aspects of wellness, including immune system function and mental health. The Mediterranean Diet's base of abundant fiber encourages the development of gut bacteria that strengthen and maintain the digestive tract.

- **Inflammation Reduction:** Chronic inflammation is a common antecedent to many chronic diseases. Because the Mediterranean Diet includes nutrients that reduce inflammation, it provides excellent resistance. Healthy meals like olive oil, fatty salmon, and a range of colorful fruits and vegetables can be taken both preventively and therapeutically. Additionally, these meals aid in lowering inflammation

The Mediterranean diet emphasizes consuming fruits, vegetables, whole grains, healthy fats, fish, poultry, and eggs on a weekly basis; consuming dairy products in moderation; and consuming red meat in moderation.

Checklist for eight scientific principles;

Principle 1: veggies

- ✓ Make an effort to consume more than two servings of vegetables every day.
- ✓ Serving size: 1 cup raw or cooked vegetables; 2 cups salad; and 1 cup raw or uncooked leafy greens
- ✓ Try a new veggie each month to add some variety to your meals.

Principle 2: Fruits and Nuts

- ✓ Aim to eat more than two servings of fruit and one serving of nuts every day.
- ✓ ½ cup dried fruit, ¼ cup fresh fruit, ¼ cup nuts, and 2 tablespoons nut butter per serving.
- ✓ Add berries and nuts to salads or cereals, and offer fruit for dessert.

Principle 3: Legume

- ✓ Change up the type of legumes you eat each week to provide some variety to your meals
- ✓ A serving is ½ cup cooked beans, peas, or lentils.
- ✓ Aim for more than two servings each week.

Principle 4: Whole Grains

- ✓ Aim to eat more than four to six meals a day.
- ✓ Portions: 7 ounces (1 ounce is equal to 1 piece of wheat bread) or 1 cup cooked grains (quinoa, brown rice, oats, etc.).
- ✓ Measure out your cereal and pasta to keep serving sizes under control.

Principle 5: Shellfish and Fish

- ✓ Aim for two or more servings of fish each week.
- ✓ A serving of 3 ounces of canned tuna and 4 ounces of fish fillet are presented.
- ✓ Fish should be seasoned with lemon juice and your favorite salt-free spice before baking.

Principle 6: Plant-Derived Fats and Oils

- ✓ In place of animal fats (butter, lard), use plant-based fats (canola oil, avocado oil, olive oil, and avocados) while cooking and eating.
- ✓ ¼ avocado and 1 TBSP olive oil each serving

✓ Mash an avocado to use as a topping for toast, potatoes, or beans; blend vinegar and olive oil to make a homemade salad dressing.

Principle 7: Dairy with Low Fat

✓ Aim for only one serving every day.
✓ The serving sizes are ¾ cup low-fat milk, 1.5 ounces natural cheese, and 6 ounces low-fat plain yogurt.
✓ Weigh cheese before adding it to recipes and use yogurt instead of mayonnaise to control portion proportions.

Principle 8: Proteins and Meats

✓ Try to limit your intake of red meat to no more than one serving per day or no more than three servings per month.
✓ Serving dimensions: One egg, three cooked chicken breast ounces, and three cooked beef tenderloin ounces. When eating, consider meat as an accompaniment rather than the main course.

<u>Health Benefits of Mediterranean Diet Backed by Research</u>

Amid the vast assortment of dietary fads, the Mediterranean Diet, with its well-researched health benefits, is a shining example of scientific confirmation. This lifestyle offers a multitude of well-established health advantages that are supported by extensive scientific study, all while satisfying the palate. It is based on the nutritional wisdom of Mediterranean civilizations.

1. **Cardiovascular Excellence:** The main health benefits of the Mediterranean diet are its notable effects on cardiovascular health. Numerous studies have shown a decreased risk of heart disease and stroke in people who follow this dietary plan. Bad cholesterol (LDL) levels are decreased and heart health is improved when omega-3 fatty acids from fatty fish and heart-healthy monounsaturated fats from olive oil are taken combined.

2. **Metabolic Harmony and Weight Management:** Changing to a Mediterranean diet is a deliberate step toward weight management. It goes beyond only taste of food. Scientific research has linked this eating habit to a lower body weight, a smaller waist circumference, and a decreased risk of obesity. In order to maintain metabolic balance and long-term weight management, it is recommended to encourage portion control, a balanced macronutrient intake, and nutrient-dense food choices.

3. **Brain Health and Cognitive Resilience:** When it comes to neurological problems associated with brain health, the Mediterranean Diet is the best option. Research suggests that living this way may lower the risk of neurological conditions including Alzheimer's and cognitive decline. Mediterranean food is rich in antioxidants, omega-3 fatty acids, and anti-inflammatory components that boost cognitive resilience by creating a neuroprotective environment.

4. **Diabetes Prevention and Management:** One effective strategy in the battle against diabetes is the Mediterranean Diet. Studies have demonstrated a link between this dietary approach and improved insulin sensitivity in addition to a lower incidence of type 2 diabetes. Due to its emphasis on whole grains, legumes, and high-fiber foods, it is a crucial approach in the prevention and management of diabetes. Blood sugar levels can be stabilized by eating these meals.

5. **Mitigation of Inflammation:** The Mediterranean Diet is also very beneficial in this regard. A lot of chronic diseases start out as chronic inflammation. Because this diet is rich in nutrients like fruits, vegetables, and olive oil that reduce inflammation, it lowers inflammation throughout the body. Scientific research backs up its capacity to reduce inflammatory markers and offer a shield against conditions like arthritis and cardiovascular disease.

6. **Longevity and overall well-being:** When talking about the health benefits of a Mediterranean diet, the subject of lifespan comes up. This eating habit has been associated in research with a longer lifespan and improved quality of life as one matures. The diet's all-encompassing strategy, along with its emphasis on social connections and meal enjoyment, encourage overall health and a more vibrant, fulfilling life.

An abundance of scientific research substantiates the health benefits of the Mediterranean Diet, painting a convincing image of a long-lasting dietary approach. In addition to being a source of sensory delight, this style of living turns out to be a powerful cure for long-term health, offering gourmet delight and scientific accuracy as trustworthy friends on the journey towards wellness.

<u>Foods to eat and foods not to eat on Mediterranean Diet</u>

Embarking on a Mediterranean diet is not only about making dietary changes; it's an exploration of flavor and health benefits supported by scientific research. To completely reap the benefits of this lifestyle and its array of wellness advantages, it becomes imperative to know which foods to eat and which to avoid.

<u>Foods to Eat:</u>

- **Fruits and vegetables:** A rainbow of colors awaits you as you feast on an abundance of fresh fruits and vegetables. These nutrient-dense delicacies are the foundation of the diet, offering a taste explosion and a multitude of health benefits. They are rich in vitamins, minerals, and antioxidants.

- **Whole Grains**: Some highly nutritious whole grains are brown rice, quinoa, and farro. These complex carbohydrates provide sustained energy, fiber, and a wealth of minerals, all of which help with overall health and weight management.

- **Fatty Fish:** Include seafood high in omega-3s, such as salmon, mackerel, and sardines, in your diet. These nutrient-dense powerhouses improve heart health, improve cognitive function, and add a tasty touch to your Mediterranean-style cuisine.

- **Legumes:** Scoop up a rainbow of beans, lentils, and chickpeas. Fiber, protein, and other nutrients that support gastrointestinal health, satiety, and weight control can all be found in abundance in legumes.

- **Nuts and Seeds**: Almonds, walnuts, and chia seeds are delicious as snacks. These nutritious additives include protein, healthy fats, and essential nutrients, making them a pleasant and nutrient-dense transition between meals.

- **Herbs and Spices:** To improve your meal, use a range of herbs and spices, such basil, oregano, and turmeric. In addition to their deliciousness, these culinary marvels include anti-inflammatory and antioxidant properties that enhance taste and health.

<u>**Foods to Avoid or Restrict:**</u>

- **Processed Foods**: Bid adieu to highly processed and refined foods. Select whole, unadulterated foods in place of artificial additives, preservatives, and additives that may offset the health benefits of the diet.

- **Added Sugars**: Get less added sugar in your diet by staying away from processed sweets, candies, and beverages with added sugar. To satisfy your sweet need, accept the natural sweetness of fruits.

- **Red and Processed Meats**: Try consuming as little red and processed meat as you can. The Mediterranean Diet allows small amounts of lean meats but stresses fish and plant-based proteins as heart-healthy alternatives.

- **Refined Grains:** Use whole grains in place of refined grains. Pick whole grains like quinoa, oats, and whole wheat to maximize nutritious value and ensure sustained energy levels.

- **Overindulgence in Dairy:** Low-fat or fermented dairy products are the best options, even if the Mediterranean Diet allows for small amounts of dairy. Cut back on high-fat dairy products to maintain a balanced, heart-healthy diet.

- **Trans Fats**: Steer clear of trans fats, which are included in many processed and fried foods. Make your daily intake of fat from foods like almonds and olive oil, which are heart-healthy alternatives.

Navigating the Mediterranean Diet is a gastronomic adventure that goes beyond nutrition; it's a celebration of flavors and a commitment to long-term health. Embrace the Mediterranean's abundance and turn each meal into a happy symphony of health and delicious food

BREAKFAST RECIPES TO ENERGIZE YOUR DAY

Greek Yogurt Parfait with Nuts and Berries

Prep Time: 5 minutes

Cooking Time: 0 minutes

Serving Size: 1

Ingredients:

- One cup of Greek yogurt
- ½ cup of mixed berries, including raspberries, blueberries, and strawberries
- One spoonful of honey
- Two tsp finely chopped nuts (walnuts, almonds)

Instructions:

1. Arrange Greek yogurt, chopped almonds, and mixed berries in a glass or dish.
2. Pour some honey on top.
3. Savor this easy breakfast that is high in protein.

Mediterranean Avocado Toast with Poached Egg.

Prep Time: 10 minutes

Cooking Time: 5 minutes

Serving Size: 1

Ingredients:

- One whole-grain piece of bread
- 1/2 mashed, ripe avocado
- One stolen egg
- To taste, add salt and pepper.
- Feta cheese and cherry tomatoes are optional.

Instruction:

1. The whole-grain bread is toasted.
2. Toast should be topped with mashed avocado.
3. Add a poached egg on top and sprinkle with salt and pepper.
4. Not required: Add some cherry tomatoes and crumbled feta as garnish.

The Fruity Mediterranean Smoothie Bowl.

Prep Time: 5 minutes

Cooking Time: 0 minutes

Serving Size: 1

Ingredients:

- One banana, frozen
- Half a cup of mixed berries
- Half a cup of Greek yogurt
- One spoonful of chia seeds
- Almond slices with granola as a garnish

Instruction:

1. Smoothly blend Greek yogurt, chia seeds, frozen banana, and mixed berries.
2. Transfer into a bowl and garnish with almond slices and granola.
3. Enjoy this nourishing and revitalizing smoothie bowl.

Mediterranean Omelette with Spinach and Feta.

Prep Time: 7 minutes

Cooking Time: 5 minutes

Serving Size: 1;

Ingredients:

- Two beaten eggs
- A handful of fresh spinach
- 1/4 cup of feta cheese, crumbled
- One tablespoon of olive oil
- To taste, add salt and pepper.

Instruction:

1. In a skillet with heated olive oil, sauté spinach until it wilts.
2. Over the spinach, pour the beaten eggs.
3. Top the omelette with feta cheese.
4. After the eggs are cooked through, fold and season.

Mediterranean Chia Seed Pudding.

Prep time: 5 minutes (plus an overnight soak)

Cooking Time: 0 minutes

Serving Size: 1

Ingredients:

- Three tsp of chia seeds
- One cup almond milk
- Half a teaspoon of extract from vanilla
- Topping: fresh berries
- A honey drizzle

Instruction:

1. In a container, combine almond milk, chia seeds, and vanilla essence.
2. Store in the fridge all night.
3. Before serving, sprinkle some honey and fresh berries over top.

Tomato and Basil Breakfast Bruschetta.

Prep Time: 10 minutes

Cooking Time: 5 minutes

Serving Size: 1

Ingredients:

- One whole-grain piece of bread
- One medium tomato, chopped
- fresh leaves of basil
- One-third cup balsamic glaze

- Use olive oil to drizzle

Instruction:

1. The whole-grain bread is toasted.
2. Add fresh basil leaves and chopped tomatoes on top.
3. Drizzle with olive oil and balsamic glaze.

Spinach and tomato frittata.

Prep Time: 10 minutes

Cooking Time: 15-minute

Serving Size: 2

Ingredients:

- Four beaten eggs
- A handful of fresh spinach
- One medium tomato, chopped
- 1/4 cup of feta cheese, crumbled
- To taste, add salt and pepper.

Instruction:

1. Set the oven's temperature to 175°C/350°F.
2. In a skillet that is oven-safe, sauté spinach until it wilts.
3. Add tomatoes, chopped, to the pan.
4. Cover the veggies with beaten eggs, top with feta, and season.
5. Bake the frittata until it sets.

Quinoa Breakfast Bowl with Almond Milk and Fresh Fruit.

Prep Time: 15 minutes

Cooking Time: 15-minute

Serving Size: 1

Ingredients:

- Half a cup of cooked quinoa
- half a cup of almond milk
- Berries and sliced banana as a topping
- 1 tablespoon of finely chopped nuts (pistachios, almonds)

Instruction:

1. Follow the directions on the package.
2. Transfer cooked quinoa to a bowl and cover with almond milk.
3. Add chopped nuts, berries, and banana slices on top.

Mediterranean Shakshuka.

Prep Time: 10 minutes

Cooking Time: 20-minute

Serving Size: 2

Ingredients:

- Four eggs
- One can, or fourteen ounces smashed tomatoes

- One chopped bell pepper
- One little onion, diced finely
- two minced garlic cloves
- One teaspoon of cumin
- One tsp of paprika
- To taste, add salt and pepper.

Instruction:

1. Bell pepper and onion should be sautéed till tender.
2. Stir in the paprika, cumin, and chopped garlic and stir until fragrant.
3. Add the smashed tomatoes, then reduce the heat for ten minutes.
4. Crack eggs into wells you've made in the sauce.
5. Cook the eggs covered until they reach your desired doneness.

Whole Grain Pancakes with Greek Yogurt and Berries.

Prep Time: 10 minutes

Cooking Time: 10 minutes

Serving Size: 2

Ingredients:

- One cup of whole grain pancake mixture
- one cup milk or water
- Greek yogurt as a garnish
- As a garnish, mixed berries

- (Optional) maple syrup

Instruction:

1. Follow the directions on the package to combine the pancake mix with milk or water.
2. Use a pan or griddle to cook pancakes.
3. Add some mixed berries and Greek yogurt over top.
4. Drizzle with maple syrup if desired.

Caprese Breakfast Sandwich

Prep Time: 10 minutes

Cooking Time: 5 minutes

Serving Size: 1

Ingredients:

- 1 whole-grain English muffin, toasted
- 1 egg, fried or poached
- 1 slice mozzarella cheese
- 1 slice tomato
- Fresh basil leaves

Instructions:

1. Toast the English muffin.
2. Assemble the sandwich with a fried or poached egg, mozzarella, tomato, and fresh basil.

<u>Fig and Walnut Overnight Oats</u>

Prep Time: 10 minutes (plus overnight soaking)

Cooking Time: 0 minutes

Serving Size: 1

Ingredients:

- 1/2 cup rolled oats
- 1/2 cup almond milk
- 2-3 fresh figs, sliced
- 1 tablespoon chopped walnuts
- Drizzle of honey

Instructions:

1. Mix rolled oats and almond milk in a jar.
2. Refrigerate overnight.
3. Top with fresh figs, chopped walnuts, and a drizzle of honey before serving.

<u>Smoked Salmon and Avocado Wrap</u>

Prep Time: 10 minutes

Cooking Time: 0 minutes

Serving Size: 1

Ingredients:

- 1 whole-grain wrap
- 2 ounces smoked salmon

- 1/2 avocado, sliced
- Handful of arugula
- Lemon wedge

Instructions:

1. Lay the whole-grain wrap flat.
2. Arrange smoked salmon, sliced avocado, and arugula on the wrap.
3. Squeeze lemon juice over the ingredients.
4. Roll the wrap and enjoy this Mediterranean-inspired delight.

Mediterranean Breakfast Burrito

Prep Time: 10 minutes

Cooking Time: 10 minutes

Serving Size: 1

Ingredients:

- 1 whole-grain tortilla
- 2 eggs, scrambled
- 1/4 cup black beans, rinsed and drained
- 1/4 cup diced tomatoes
- 1 tablespoon chopped fresh cilantro
- Salsa for topping

Instructions:

1. Heat the whole-grain tortilla.

2. Fill the tortilla with scrambled eggs, black beans, diced tomatoes, and cilantro.
3. Top with salsa.

Mediterranean Breakfast Quinoa Bowl

Prep Time: 15 minutes

Cooking Time: 15 minutes

Serving Size: 1

Ingredients:

- 1/2 cup cooked quinoa
- 1/4 cup hummus
- Cherry tomatoes, halved
- Cucumber slices
- Kalamata olives

Instructions:

1. Cook quinoa according to package instructions.
2. In a bowl, layer cooked quinoa with hummus, cherry tomatoes, cucumber slices, and Kalamata olives.

Breakfast Stuffed Bell Peppers

Prep Time: 15 minutes

Cooking Time: 20 minutes

Serving Size: 2

Ingredients:

- 2 large bell peppers, halved
- 4 eggs
- Spinach, chopped
- Feta cheese, crumbled
- Salt and pepper to taste

Instructions:

1. Preheat the oven to 375°F (190°C).
2. Hollow out bell peppers and place them on a baking sheet.
3. In each side of the bell pepper, crack an egg.
4. Add chopped spinach and crumbled feta.
5. Bake until the eggs are set.

Lemon Ricotta Pancakes with Fresh Berries

Prep Time: 15 minutes

Cooking Time: 10 minutes

Serving Size: 2

Ingredients:

- 1 cup ricotta cheese
- 2 large eggs
- 1/2 cup whole wheat flour
- 1/2 teaspoon baking powder
- Zest of 1 lemon
- Fresh berries for topping

Instructions:

1. In a bowl, mix ricotta cheese, eggs, flour, baking powder, and lemon zest.
2. Cook pancakes on a griddle or pan.
3. Top with fresh berries.

Mediterranean Breakfast Pizza

Prep Time: 10 minutes

Cooking Time: 15 minutes

Serving Size: 2

Ingredients:

- 2 whole-grain pitas
- 4 eggs
- 1/2 cup cherry tomatoes, sliced
- 1/4 cup feta cheese, crumbled
- Fresh basil leaves

Instructions:

1. Preheat the oven to 400°F (200°C).
2. Place whole-grain pitas on a baking sheet.
3. Crack eggs onto the pitas and add sliced cherry tomatoes.
4. Bake until eggs are set, then sprinkle with crumbled feta and fresh basil.

Green Shakshuka with Kale and Zucchini

Prep Time: 10 minutes

Cooking Time: 15 minutes

Serving Size: 2

Ingredients:

- 4 eggs
- 1 bunch kale, chopped
- 1 zucchini, diced
- 1 onion, finely chopped
- 2 cloves garlic, minced
- 1 teaspoon cumin
- 1 teaspoon paprika
- Salt and pepper to taste

Instructions:

1. Sauté onion and garlic until softened.
2. Add kale and zucchini, cook until vegetables are tender.
3. Season with cumin, paprika, salt, and pepper.
4. In the mixture, create wells and crack eggs into them.
5. Cook the eggs covered until they reach your desired doneness.

Almond and Berry Breakfast Couscous

Prep Time: 10 minutes

Cooking Time: 5 minutes

Serving Size: 2

Ingredients:

- 1 cup cooked couscous

- 1/4 cup almond butter
- Mixed berries for topping
- Drizzle of honey

Instructions:

1. In a bowl, mix cooked couscous with almond butter.
2. Add some mixed berries and a honey drizzle over top.
3. Stir until the almond butter is evenly distributed, creating a creamy texture throughout the couscous.
4. Divide the almond and berry-infused couscous into serving bowls.
5. Garnish generously with an assortment of fresh berries.
6. Drizzle a touch of honey over the top for a delightful sweetness.

Serve this nutrient-packed and energizing breakfast couscous, savoring the harmonious blend of flavors.

Serve this nutrient-packed and energizing breakfast couscous, savoring the harmonious blend of flavors.

LAUNCH RECIPES FOR BUSY AFTERNOONS

Greek Chickpea Salad Wrap

Prep Time: 10 minutes

Cooking Time: 0 minutes

Serving Size: 1

Ingredients:

- 1 whole-grain wrap
- 1 cup canned chickpeas, drained and rinsed
- 1/2 cucumber, diced
- 1/4 cup cherry tomatoes, halved
- 2 tbsp feta cheese, crumbled
- 1 tbsp olive oil
- 1 tsp lemon juice
- Salt and pepper to taste

Instructions:

1. In a bowl, mix chickpeas, cucumber, tomatoes, and feta.
2. Drizzle olive oil and lemon juice over the mixture.
3. Season with salt and pepper.
4. Spoon the mixture onto a whole-grain wrap, fold, and enjoy!

Mediterranean Quinoa Bowl

Prep Time: 15 minutes

Cooking Time: 15 minutes

Serving Size: 2

Ingredients:

- 1 cup cooked quinoa
- 1/2 cup cherry tomatoes, halved
- 1/2 cup cucumber, diced
- 1/4 cup Kalamata olives, sliced
- 1/4 cup red onion, finely chopped
- 1/4 cup crumbled feta cheese
- 2 tbsp olive oil
- Fresh oregano for garnish

Instructions:

1. Mix quinoa, tomatoes, cucumber, olives, red onion, and feta in a bowl.
2. Drizzle with olive oil and toss gently.
3. Garnish with fresh oregano before serving.

<u>Lemon Garlic Shrimp Skewers</u>

Prep Time: 10 minutes

Cooking Time: 5 minutes

Serving Size: 2

Ingredients:

1. 12 large shrimp, peeled and deveined

2. 2 tbsp olive oil
3. 2 cloves garlic, minced
4. 1 tsp lemon zest
5. 1 tbsp lemon juice
6. 1 tsp dried oregano
7. Salt and pepper to taste

Instructions:

1. In a bowl, mix olive oil, garlic, lemon zest, lemon juice, oregano, salt, and pepper.
2. Thread shrimp onto skewers.
3. Brush the shrimp with the lemon-garlic mixture.
4. Grill for 2-3 minutes per side until cooked through.

Greek Salad Stuffed Avocado

Prep Time: 15 minutes

Cooking Time: 0 minutes

Serving Size: 1

Ingredients:

- 1 ripe avocado, halved and pitted
- 1 cup cherry tomatoes, halved
- 1/2 cucumber, diced
- 1/4 cup red onion, finely chopped
- 1/4 cup crumbled feta cheese
- 2 tbsp Kalamata olives, sliced
- 1 tbsp olive oil

- 1 tsp red wine vinegar
- Salt and pepper to taste

Instructions:

1. In a bowl, mix tomatoes, cucumber, red onion, feta, and olives.
2. Olive oil and red wine vinegar should be drizzled on, then gently mixed.
3. Spoon the salad into avocado halves, and season with salt and pepper.

Mediterranean Hummus and Veggie Wrap

Prep Time: 10 minutes

Cooking Time: 0 minutes

Serving Size: 1

Ingredients:

- 1 whole-grain wrap
- 1/4 cup hummus
- 1/2 cup mixed bell peppers, sliced
- 1/2 cup cucumber, julienned
- 1/4 cup red onion, thinly sliced
- 1/4 cup cherry tomatoes, halved
- Fresh parsley for garnish

Instructions:

- Spread hummus evenly on the whole-grain wrap.

- Layer the wrap with bell peppers, cucumber, red onion, and cherry tomatoes.
- Garnish with fresh parsley before rolling it up.

Lemon Herb Grilled Chicken Salad

Prep Time: 15 minutes

Cooking Time: 10 minutes

Serving Size: 2

Ingredients:

- 2 boneless, skinless chicken breasts
- 2 tbsp olive oil
- 2 cloves garlic, minced
- 1 tsp dried oregano
- Zest of 1 lemon
- 2 tbsp lemon juice
- Salt and pepper to taste
- Mixed greens for the salad

Instructions:

1. In a bowl, mix olive oil, garlic, oregano, lemon zest, lemon juice, salt, and pepper.
2. Coat chicken breasts with the marinade and grill for 4-5 minutes per side.
3. Slice chicken and serve over a bed of mixed greens.

Mediterranean Egg Salad Lettuce Wraps

Prep Time: 10 minutes

Cooking Time: 10 minutes

Serving Size: 2

Ingredients:

- 4 hard-boiled eggs, chopped
- 1/4 cup cucumber, diced
- 1/4 cup cherry tomatoes, halved
- 2 tbsp Kalamata olives, sliced
- 2 tbsp red onion, finely chopped
- 2 tbsp Greek yogurt
- 1 tbsp Dijon mustard
- Salt and pepper to taste
- Butter lettuce leaves for wrapping

Instructions:

1. In a bowl, mix eggs, cucumber, tomatoes, olives, and red onion.
2. Stir in Greek yogurt and Dijon mustard.
3. Season with salt and pepper, and spoon into lettuce leaves.

Tomato Basil Mozzarella Skewers

Prep Time: 10 minutes

Cooking Time: 0 minutes

Serving Size: 2

Ingredients:

- 16 cherry tomatoes
- 8 fresh mozzarella balls
- Fresh basil leaves
- 2 tbsp balsamic glaze
- Salt and pepper to taste

Instructions:

1. Thread cherry tomatoes, mozzarella, and basil onto skewers.
2. Add a balsamic glaze drizzle and season with salt and pepper.

Zucchini and Feta Fritters

Prep Time: 15 minutes

Cooking Time: 10 minutes

Serving Size: 2

Ingredients:

- 2 medium zucchinis, grated
- 1/4 cup feta cheese, crumbled
- 2 tbsp fresh mint, chopped
- 1 egg
- 2 tbsp whole wheat flour
- 2 tbsp olive oil
- Greek yogurt for dipping

Instructions:

1. Squeeze excess water from grated zucchini.

2. In a bowl, mix zucchini, feta, mint, egg, and flour.
3. Form into patties and pan-fry in olive oil until golden.
4. Pair with Greek yogurt for dipping.

Shrimp and Spinach Greek Quesadilla

Prep Time: 10 minutes

Cooking Time: 5 minutes

Serving Size: 1

Ingredients:

- 2 whole-grain tortillas
- 6 large shrimp, peeled and deveined
- Handful of fresh spinach
- 1/4 cup feta cheese, crumbled
- 2 tbsp sun-dried tomatoes, chopped
- 1 tbsp olive oil

Instructions:

1. Heat olive oil and sauté prawns till done.
2. On a tortilla, layer spinach, shrimp, feta, and sun-dried tomatoes.
3. Top with the second tortilla and grill until cheese melts.

Greek Lemon Chicken Pita Pockets

Prep Time: 15 minutes

Cooking Time: 15 minutes

Serving Size: 2

Ingredients:

- 2 boneless, skinless chicken breasts
- 1 lemon, juiced and zested
- 2 cloves garlic, minced
- 1 tsp dried oregano
- Salt and pepper to taste
- 2 whole-grain pita pockets
- 1/2 cup Greek yogurt
- 1/4 cup cucumber, diced

Instructions:

1. Marinate chicken in lemon juice, lemon zest, garlic, oregano, salt, and pepper.
2. Grill until cooked through and slice.
3. Stuff pita pockets with chicken, Greek yogurt, and diced cucumber.

Spinach and Feta Stuffed Chicken Breast

Prep Time: 15 minutes

Cooking Time: 25 minutes

Serving Size: 2

Ingredients:

- 2 boneless, skinless chicken breasts
- 2 cups fresh spinach, chopped

- 1/4 cup feta cheese, crumbled
- 2 cloves garlic, minced
- 1 tsp dried oregano
- Salt and pepper to taste
- Instructions:
- Preheat oven to 375°F (190°C).
- Mix spinach, feta, garlic, oregano, salt, and pepper.
- Cut a pocket into each chicken breast and stuff with the spinach mixture.
- Bake until chicken is done, 20–25 minutes.

Greek Yogurt Berry Parfait

Prep Time: 5 minutes

Cooking Time: 0 minutes

Serving Size: 1

Ingredients:

1 cup Greek yogurt

1/2 cup mixed berries (strawberries, blueberries, raspberries)

2 tbsp honey

2 tbsp granola

Instructions:

1. In a glass, layer Greek yogurt, berries, and granola.
2. Drizzle with honey before serving.

Mediterranean Tuna Salad

Prep Time: 10 minutes

Cooking Time: 0 minutes

Serving Size: 2

Ingredients:

- 2 cans tuna, drained
- 1/2 cup cherry tomatoes, halved
- 1/4 cup red onion, finely chopped
- 2 tbsp Kalamata olives, sliced
- 2 tbsp olive oil
- 1 tbsp red wine vinegar
- Salt and pepper to taste

Instructions:

1. In a bowl, mix tuna, tomatoes, red onion, and olives.
2. Drizzle with olive oil and red wine vinegar.
3. Season with salt and pepper before serving.

Roasted Vegetable Couscous Bowl

Prep Time: 15 minutes

Cooking Time: 20 minutes

Serving Size: 2

Ingredients:

- 1 cup whole wheat couscous, cooked

- 1 zucchini, sliced
- 1 red bell pepper, sliced
- 1/2 red onion, sliced
- 2 tbsp olive oil
- 1 tsp dried thyme
- Salt and pepper to taste

Instructions:

1. Preheat oven to 400°F (200°C).
2. Toss zucchini, bell pepper, and red onion in olive oil and thyme.
3. Roast veggies for 20 minutes to soften.
4. Serve over cooked whole wheat couscous.

DINNER RECIPES FOR DELICIOUS EVENINGS

Grilled chicken salad with Mediterranean flavors

Prep Time: 15 minutes

Cooking Time: 15-minute

2 serving size

Ingredients

- One skinless and boneless chicken breast
- two cups of mixed greens
- Half a cup of cherry tomatoes
- 1/4 cup pitted Kalamata olives, 1 cucumber, 1/4 cup crumbled Feta cheese
- Two teaspoons pure olive oil
- One-third cup balsamic vinegar
- To taste, add salt and pepper.

Instructions

1. After adding salt and pepper to the chicken breast, broil it until it is cooked through.
2. Mix the mixed greens, cucumber, cherry tomatoes, olives, and feta cheese in a big bowl.
3. Arrange the grilled chicken slices over the salad.
4. Mix the balsamic vinegar and olive oil in a small bowl. Pour over the greens.

Stuffed Bell Peppers with Quinoa

Prep Time: 20 minutes

Cooking Time: 30 minutes

4 serving size

Ingredients:

- One cup cooked quinoa, four halved bell peppers with seeds removed
- Quinoa, washed and drained, in one can (15 oz).
- One cup diced cherry tomatoes, half a cup crumbled feta cheese, two teaspoons minced fresh parsley, and one tablespoon olive oil
- One teaspoon of cumin powder
- To taste, add salt and pepper.

Instructions

1. Preheat the oven to 375°F, or 190°C.
2. Combine the cooked quinoa, chickpeas, feta cheese, cherry tomatoes, parsley, cumin, olive oil, and salt and pepper in a bowl.
3. Stuff the quinoa mixture into each side of a bell pepper.
4. After placing the filled peppers on a baking tray, bake them for thirty minutes, or until they become soft.

Pasta with Lemon Garlic Shrimp

Prep Time: 10 minutes

Cooking Time: 15-minute

2 serving size

Ingredients:

- Eight-ounce whole-wheat spaghetti
- Half a pound of shrimp, peeled and deveined; three garlic cloves, chopped; one lemon, squeezed and zest
- Two tsp olive oil
- 1/4 cup finely chopped fresh parsley
- To taste, add salt and pepper.
- grating Parmesan cheese (not required)

Instructions

1. Follow the directions.
2. Warm up some olive oil in a pan over medium heat. When aromatic, add the minced garlic and sauté it.
3. Cook the prawns in the pan until they become pink.
4. Add shrimp, lemon zest, juice, parsley, salt, and pepper to cooked pasta and toss.
5. Not required: Before serving, top with grated Parmesan cheese.

<u>Mediterranean Vegetable Baked Salmon</u>

Prep Time: 15 minutes

Cooking Time: 25-minute

2 serving size

Ingredients:

- Two fillets of salmon

- One bell pepper, one sliced red onion, and one sliced zucchini
- One cup of cherry tomatoes
- Two tsp olive oil
- Two tsp of dry oregano
- To taste, add salt and pepper.
- slices of lemon for serving

Instructions

1. Set oven temperature to 400°F, or 200°C.
2. Salmon fillets should be put on a baking pan.
3. Combine the cherry tomatoes, bell pepper, red onion, and zucchini in a bowl and mix with the olive oil, oregano, salt, and pepper.
4. On the baking sheet, arrange the veggies around the salmon.
5. Bake for 25 minutes, or until the veggies are soft and the salmon is cooked through. Accompany with slices of lemon.

Turkey Burgers with Greek Flavor

Prep Time: 20 minutes

Cooking Time: 15-minute

4 serving size

Ingredients

- One pound of ground turkey
- half a cup of breadcrumbs made with whole wheat

- 1/4 cup of coarsely chopped red onion
- 1/4 cup of crumbled feta cheese
- 1/4 cup finely minced black olives
- Two tsp of dry oregano
- one tsp powdered garlic
- To taste, add salt and pepper.
- Burger buns made entirely of wheat
- Tzatziki dressing as a garnish

Instructions

1. Ground turkey, breadcrumbs, feta cheese, red onion, black olives, oregano, garlic powder, salt, and pepper should all be combined in a dish.
2. Create patties out of the mixture.
3. The turkey burgers should be cooked through on a stovetop or grill.
4. Serve with tzatziki sauce on top of whole wheat bread.

Eggplant and Chickpea Stew

Prep Time: 15 minutes

Cooking Time: 30 minutes

Serving Size: 4

Ingredients:

- 1 large eggplant, diced
- 1 can (15 oz) chickpeas, drained and rinsed
- 1 onion, diced

- 2 cloves garlic, minced
- 1 can (14 oz) diced tomatoes
- 1 teaspoon ground cumin
- 1 teaspoon paprika
- 1/2 teaspoon ground cinnamon
- 2 tablespoons olive oil
- Fresh parsley for garnish
- Salt and pepper to taste

Instructions:

1. Warm up the olive oil in a big saucepan over medium heat. Add diced onion and sauté until translucent.
2. Add minced garlic, ground cumin, paprika, and ground cinnamon. Stir for 1-2 minutes.
3. Add diced eggplant, chickpeas, and diced tomatoes with their juices. Season with salt and pepper.
4. Cover and simmer for 25-30 minutes, stirring occasionally.
5. Garnish with fresh parsley before serving.

Mediterranean Cauliflower Rice Bowl

Prep Time: 10 minutes

Cooking Time: 15 minutes

Serving Size: 2

Ingredients:

- 1 cauliflower, grated into rice
- 1 cup cherry tomatoes, halved

- 1/2 cucumber, diced
- 1/4 cup Kalamata olives, pitted and sliced
- 1/4 cup feta cheese, crumbled
- 2 tablespoons olive oil
- 1 tablespoon red wine vinegar
- 1 teaspoon dried oregano
- Salt and pepper to taste
- Grilled chicken or chickpeas for protein (optional)

Instructions:

1. In a large pan, sauté cauliflower rice in olive oil until tender.
2. In a bowl, combine cauliflower rice, cherry tomatoes, cucumber, olives, and feta cheese.
3. Olive oil, red wine vinegar, dried oregano, salt, and pepper ought to be mixed in a small dish. Drizzle over the cauliflower rice mixture.
4. Optional: Top with grilled chicken or chickpeas for added protein.

Lemon Herb Baked Cod

Prep Time: 10 minutes

Cooking Time: 20 minutes

Serving Size: 2

Ingredients:

- 2 cod fillets
- 1 lemon, sliced

- 2 tablespoons fresh parsley, chopped
- 1 tablespoon olive oil
- 1 teaspoon dried thyme
- 1 teaspoon garlic powder
- Salt and pepper to taste

Instructions:

1. Preheat the oven to 375°F (190°C).
2. Place cod fillets on a baking sheet.
3. Drizzle olive oil over the cod and season with dried thyme, garlic powder, salt, and pepper.
4. Add a slice of lemon over each fillet.
5. Bake for 20 minutes or until the cod is flaky. Garnish with fresh parsley before serving.

Spinach and Feta Stuffed Chicken Breast

Prep Time: 15 minutes

Cooking Time: 25 minutes

Serving Size: 2

Ingredients:

- 2 boneless, skinless chicken breasts
- 2 cups fresh spinach, chopped
- 1/4 cup feta cheese, crumbled
- 1/4 cup sun-dried tomatoes, chopped
- 1 tablespoon olive oil
- 1 teaspoon dried oregano

- Salt and pepper to taste

Instructions:

1. Preheat the oven to 375°F (190°C).
2. In a pan, sauté chopped spinach in olive oil until wilted. Remove from heat.
3. Butterfly each chicken breast and fill with sautéed spinach, feta cheese, and sun-dried tomatoes.
4. Sprinkle dried oregano, salt, and pepper on each stuffed chicken breast.
5. Bake the chicken for 25 minutes, or until it is well done.

Greek Lentil Soup

Prep Time: 15 minutes

Cooking Time: 30 minutes

Serving Size: 4

Ingredients:

- 1 cup dry green lentils, rinsed
- 1 onion, diced
- 2 carrots, diced
- 2 celery stalks, diced
- 3 cloves garlic, minced
- 1 can (14 oz) diced tomatoes
- 6 cups vegetable broth
- 1 teaspoon dried oregano
- 1 teaspoon ground cumin

- 2 tablespoons olive oil
- Fresh lemon wedges for serving
- Salt and pepper to taste

Instructions:

1. Warm up the olive oil in a big saucepan over medium heat. Add diced onion, carrots, and celery. Sauté until vegetables are softened.
2. Add minced garlic, dried oregano, and ground cumin. Stir for 1-2 minutes.
3. Add lentils, diced tomatoes, and vegetable broth. Season with salt and pepper.
4. Bring the soup to a boil, then reduce heat and simmer for 25-30 minutes or until lentils are tender.
5. Serve with a squeeze of fresh lemon.

Enjoy these delicious and nutritious Mediterranean dinner recipes for flavorful evenings that contribute to your health and weight loss journey!

SNACK AND SIDES

A plate of Mediterranean hummus

Prep Time: 10 minutes

Cooking Time: 0 minutes

1 serving size

Ingredients:

- Half a cup of hummus
- One cup cherry tomatoes, one-half cucumber, one-fourth cup Kalamata olives, one tablespoon extra-virgin olive oil, and one pit
- one tsp lemon juice
- To taste, add salt and pepper.

Instructions

1. Place the hummus in the middle of the platter.
2. Arrange cucumber slices, cherry tomatoes, and Kalamata olives around the hummus.
3. Pour in some lemon juice and olive oil.
4. To taste, add salt and pepper for seasoning.
5. Savor with veggie sticks or whole-grain pita.

Dip of Greek Yogurt Tzatziki

Prep Time: 15 minutes

Cooking Time: 0 minutes

2 serving size

Ingredients:

1. One cup of Greek yogurt
2. Grate half of a cucumber and mince two garlic cloves.
3. One tablespoon finely chopped fresh dill and one tablespoon of extra virgin olive oil
4. To taste, add salt and pepper.

Instructions

1. In a bowl, mix Greek yogurt, chopped dill, minced garlic, and shredded cucumber.
2. Pour in some olive oil and stir thoroughly.
3. To taste, add salt and pepper for seasoning.
4. Before serving, let the food cool for at least half an hour in the refrigerator.
5. Accompany with whole-grain crackers or carrot sticks.

Stuffed Grape Leaves in the Mediterranean

Prep Time: 20 minutes

Cooking Time: 0 minutes

4 serving size

Ingredients:

- One cup of drained canned grape leaves
- One cup of cooked quinoa

- 1/2 cup diced cherry tomatoes, 1/4 cup crumbled feta cheese, 2 tablespoons minced fresh mint, and 1 tablespoon extra-virgin olive oil
- slices of lemon for serving

Instructions

1. Combine the cooked quinoa, feta cheese, chopped mint, and diced cherry tomatoes in a bowl.
2. Arrange the grape leaves and stuff the quinoa mixture into each one.
3. Pour some olive oil over it.
4. Accompany with slices of lemon.

Salad with Mediterranean Chickpeas

Prep Time: 15 minutes

Cooking Time: 0 minutes

2 serving size

Ingredients:

- One 15-ounce can of well washed and drained beans
- Half a cup of cherry tomatoes
- 1/4 cup of coarsely chopped red onion
- 1/4 cup of crumbled feta cheese
- Two teaspoons of freshly chopped parsley
- One tablespoon of extra virgin olive oil
- One tablespoon of vinegar made from red wine
- To taste, add salt and pepper.

Instructions

1. Chickpeas, cherry tomatoes, red onion, feta cheese, and parsley should all be combined in a bowl.
2. Add a drizzle of red wine vinegar and olive oil.
3. To taste, add salt and pepper for seasoning.
4. Before serving, toss thoroughly and chill for at least half an hour.

<u>Roasted Red Pepper Hummus from the Mediterranean</u>

Prep Time: 10 minutes

Cooking Time: 20 minutes (including roasting time)

4 serving size

Ingredients:

- One 15-ounce can of well washed and drained beans
- Roasted red peppers, half a cup
- 1/4 cup tahini and 2 garlic cloves
- two tsp lemon juice
- Two teaspoons pure olive oil
- To taste, add cayenne and salt.

Instructions

1. Put the tahini, garlic, lemon juice, roasted red peppers, and chickpeas in a food processor.
2. Olive oil is added gradually while blending until smooth.
3. To taste, add cayenne and salt for seasoning.

4.   Accompany with slices of cucumber or whole-grain pita.

Skewers with Mediterranean Caprese

Prep Time: 15 minutes

Cooking Time: 0 minutes

4 serving size

Ingredients:

- One cup of cherry tomatoes
- One cup of freshly made mozzarella sticks
- fresh leaves of basil
- Drizzling toothpicks with balsamic glaze

Instructions

1.   On each toothpick, thread a cherry tomato, a mozzarella ball, and a basil leaf.
2.   Place the skewers in a serving plate arrangement.
3.   Before serving, drizzle with balsamic glaze.

Feta and Zucchini Fritters

Prep Time: 20 minutes

Cooking Time: 10 minutes

3 serving size

Ingredients:

- Grated two medium zucchini and crumbled half a cup of feta cheese
- One-fourth cup of whole wheat flour
- One egg
- Two teaspoons of freshly chopped dill
- To taste, add salt and pepper.
- Use olive oil for cooking.

Instructions

1. Grated zucchini, feta cheese, whole wheat flour, egg, and chopped dill should all be combined in a bowl.
2. To taste, add salt and pepper for seasoning.
3. In a pan over medium heat, warm the olive oil.
4. To make little fritters, spoon ingredients into pan.
5. Cook till golden brown, 3–4 minutes on each side.

Cucumber Salad Mediterranean Style

Prep Time: 15 minutes

Cooking Time: 0 minutes

2 serving size

Ingredients:

- One cucumber, cut thinly
- Half a cup of cherry tomatoes
- 1/4 cup finely sliced red onion, 2 tablespoons crumbled feta cheese
- A tablespoon of finely chopped fresh mint and a tablespoon of extra virgin olive oil

- One tablespoon of vinegar made from red wine
- To taste, add salt and pepper.

Instructions

1. Cucumber slices, cherry tomatoes, red onion, feta cheese, and mint should all be combined in a bowl.
2. Add a drizzle of red wine vinegar and olive oil.
3. To taste, add salt and pepper for seasoning.
4. Before serving, gently toss and chill for at least half an hour.

Cups of Mediterranean Quinoa Salad

Prep Time: 20 minutes

Quinoa Cooking Time: 15 Minutes

4 serving size

Ingredients:

- One cup of cooked quinoa
- 1/2 cup chopped cucumber, 1/2 cup diced cherry tomatoes, 1/4 cup quartered red bell pepper, diced 2 tablespoons chopped feta cheese, 2 tablespoons chopped Kalamata olives, 1 tablespoon chopped fresh parsley, and 1 tablespoon chopped extra virgin olive oil
- slices of lemon for serving
- For cups, use Bibb lettuce leaves.

Instructions

1. The cooked quinoa, cucumber, cherry tomatoes, red bell pepper, feta cheese, Kalamata olives, and parsley should all be combined in a dish.
2. Give it a little toss and drizzle with olive oil.
3. To make cups, spoon the quinoa salad into the Bibb lettuce leaves.
4. Accompany with slices of lemon.

Roasted Eggplant Dip from the Mediterranean

Prep Time: 15 minutes

Cooking Time: 30 minutes (including roasting time)

4 serving size

Ingredients:

- One huge eggplant
- two garlic cloves
- Twice as much tahini
- Two teaspoons pure olive oil
- One tablespoon of lemon juice
- One tablespoon of freshly chopped parsley
- To taste, add cayenne and salt.
- Pita made with whole grains to serve

Instructions

1. Set oven temperature to 400°F, or 200°C.
2. Using a fork, pierce the eggplant and transfer it to a baking pan.

3. Roast until the meat is tender and the skin is browned, about 25 to 30 minutes.
4. After letting the eggplant cool, cut and peel its flesh.
5. Combine the eggplant, garlic, tahini, olive oil, lemon juice, chopped parsley, salt, and cayenne pepper in a food processor and pulse until smooth.
6. Present with wholegrain pita.

These side dish and snack dishes with Mediterranean influences will not only tempt your palate but also help you on your path to a better way of living. Savor these delicious dishes while providing your body with the healthful benefits of a Mediterranean diet.

DESSERTS AND SWEET INDULGENCES

Greek Yogurt and Fresh Berry Parfait

Prep Time: 5 minutes

Cooking Time: 0 minutes

1 serving size

Ingredients:

- One cup of Greek yogurt
- ½ cup of mixed berries, including raspberries, blueberries, and strawberries
- One spoonful of honey
- 1 tablespoon of finely chopped nuts (walnuts or almonds)

Instructions

1. Arrange Greek yogurt layers in a glass or dish.
2. Add a mixture of berries on top.
3. Pour honey on top of the fruit.
4. Add some chopped nuts on the top.
5. If desired, repeat the layers.
6. Present cold.

Apples Baked with Walnuts and Cinnamon

Prep Time: 10 minutes

Cooking Time: 25-minute

2 serving size

Ingredients:

- 2 apples, cut in half and cored
- One tsp of cinnamon
- two teaspoons of finely chopped walnuts
- One spoonful of honey

Instructions

1. Set the oven to 190°C, or 375°F.
2. Apple halves should be put on a baking pan.
3. Dredge the apples with cinnamon.
4. Add chopped walnuts to the apple cores.
5. Pour some honey on top.
6. Bake the apples for 25 minutes, or until they are soft.
7. Warm up and serve.

<u>Strawberries Dipped in Dark Chocolate.</u>

Prep Time: 10 minutes

Cooking time: 1 minute

4 serving size

Ingredients:

- One cup of fresh, dried and cleaned strawberries
- One-fourth cup of dark chocolate chips
- One tsp of coconut oil

Instructions

- Melt dark chocolate chips and coconut oil in a basin that is safe to microwave for 20 seconds at a time, stirring in between.
- Each strawberry should be dipped in the melted chocolate.
- Spoon onto a tray coated with paper.
- Let the chocolate harden.
- Present cold.
- Prep Time: 15 minutes for Orange and Almond Cake
- 30 minutes Cooking Time
- 8-ounce Serving Size

Ingredients:

- two cups of almond flour
- One cup of Greek yogurt
- Three big eggs
- half a cup of honey
- One orange's zest
- One tsp baking powder

Instructions:

1. Add a pinch of salt.
2. Set the oven's temperature to 175°C/350°F.
3. Almond flour, Greek yogurt, eggs, honey, orange zest, baking powder, and salt should all be well mixed in a basin.
4. Fill a cake pan that has been oiled with batter.
5. Remove the toothpick after 30 minutes of baking.
6. Let cool completely before slicing.
7. Allow to settle at room temperature.

Mint-infused Mediterranean Fruit Salad

Prep Time: 10 minutes

Cooking Time: 0 minutes

4 serving size

Ingredients:

- One cup diced watermelon, one cup diced cantaloupe, one cup diced grapes, one cup fresh mint leaves, chopped, and one tablespoon honey
- One lemon's juice

Instructions

1. Put the grapes, cantaloupe, and watermelon in a big dish.
2. Whisk the lemon juice and honey together in a small bowl.
3. Over the fruit, drizzle the honey-lemon mixture.
4. Toss lightly to blend after adding the chopped mint.
5. Present cold.

Almond and Fig Bites

Prep Time: 15 minutes

Cooking Time: 0 minutes

Serving Size: 6

Ingredients:

- Twelve dehydrated figs
- half a cup of almond butter

- 1/4 cup of coconut, shredded

Instructions

- Cut desiccated figs in half.
- Take each fig half and spread one side with almond butter.
- Two halves may be pressed together to form a "sandwich."
- Coat the edges with coconut shreds.
- Continue with the remaining figs.
- Allow to settle at room temperature.

Mango-Chia Seed Pudding

Prep time: 5 minutes (plus cooling time)

Cooking Time: 0 minutes

2 serving size

Ingredients:

- One-fourth cup chia seeds
- One cup almond milk
- One tsp vanilla essence
- One spoonful of honey
- One ripe mango, chopped

Instructions

1. Mix the almond milk, honey, vanilla essence, and chia seeds in a bowl.
2. Stir periodically and refrigerate for at least two hours or overnight.

3. Arrange the chopped mango and chia pudding in serving glasses after the mixture has thickened.
4. Present cold.

Frozen Bits with Yogurt and Pistachios

Prep Time: 10 minutes

Cooking Time: 0 minutes (freezing time)

Serving Size: 6

Ingredients:

- One cup of Greek yogurt
- 1/4 cup of pistachios, chopped
- two tsp honey

Instructions

1. Combine Greek yogurt, honey, and chopped pistachios in a bowl.
2. Pour the mixture into ice cube trays or silicone molds using a spoon.
3. Freeze until it solidifies.
4. After removing the frozen bits from the molds, serve them.

Orange Blossom Water Cookies with Almonds

Prep Time: 15 minutes

Cooking Time: 12 minutes

12 serving size

Ingredients:

- One cup of almond flour
- 1/4 cup of honey
- One egg
- One tsp orange blossom water
- One orange's zest

Instructions

1. Set the oven's temperature to 175°C/350°F.
2. Almond flour, honey, egg, orange blossom water, and orange zest should all be combined in a bowl to make dough.
3. Transfer amounts the size of a tablespoon onto a baking sheet.
4. Bake until the edges become brown, about 12 minutes.
5. Let cool completely before serving.

<u>Oatmeal and Berry Crumble</u>

Prep Time: 10 minutes

Cooking Time: 25-minute

Serving Size: 6

Ingredients:

- Two cups of mixed berries, including raspberries, blueberries, and strawberries
- One cup of traditional oats

- One-fourth cup almond flour
- two tsp honey
- Two teaspoons of melted coconut oil

Instructions

1. Set the oven's temperature to 175°C/350°F.
2. Combine berries and honey in a basin, then transfer to a baking dish.
3. To prepare the crumble topping, mix oats, almond flour, and melted coconut oil in a separate dish.
4. Scatter the crumble evenly over the fruit.
5. Bake for 25 minutes, or until the berries are bubbling and the top is brown.
6. Warm up and serve.

These delightfully balanced sweets with Mediterranean influences are ideal for anybody trying to cut weight and lead a healthy lifestyle. Savor these pleasures that honor the richness of the Mediterranean diet without feeling guilty.

CONCLUSION

As we flip the last page of the "Mediterranean Diet Meal Prep and Recipes Cookbook for Beginners," we are embarking on a lifestyle change in addition to wrapping up a culinary adventure. This collection of recipes has been more than just a guide; it has been a journey partner on your journey to wellness, offering a taste of the nutritious meals, variety of flavors, and traditional wisdom of the Mediterranean.

You've learned the importance of eating simply, how to savor every bite, and how maintaining a balanced diet may enhance your general health with these dishes. All of the meals, including the dessert, have been carefully prepared with your health and wellness in mind.

As you reflect on the pages you've turned and the meals you've enjoyed, keep in mind that the Mediterranean diet is a way of life rather than merely a set of guidelines. It's about embracing a journey to become a better version of yourself, savoring the beauty of freshly prepared food, and spending time with loved ones during mealtimes

There's a universe of delectable possibilities outside the cookbook. Continue playing around with these recipes, adding your own touches to make each dish appear like you. Let the Mediterranean diet be more than just one chapter in your life; let it be a constant source of joy, peace, and nourishment.

With any luck, this cookbook will serve as a constant source of inspiration for you, guiding you in creating dishes that will please both your palate and your overall health. Put the book down and consider it as a gateway to a lifestyle full of mindful eating, healthy choices, and the delight of savoring every moment.

We are grateful that you have welcomed these recipes into your kitchen and home. We toast to a happy, healthier you in the future, filled with delectable dishes and well-balanced meals!

BONUS MATERIALS (3 GIFTS)

1st GIFT: Mediterranean Diet Grocery Shopping List

Beginning a Mediterranean diet is not just a commitment to eating healthily but also a celebration of flavors, colors, and a lifestyle built on nourishing food. This meticulously designed grocery shopping list will help you fill your basket with vibrant, nutrient-dense jewels while navigating the world of Mediterranean-inspired culinary adventures.

Fruits and Vegetables:

- Tomatoes
- Spinach
- Kale
- Bell peppers
- Eggplant
- Zucchini
- Avocados
- Oranges
- Berries (strawberries, blueberries, raspberries)
- Lemons

Whole Grains:

- Quinoa
- Farro
- Brown rice

- Bulgur
- Whole wheat couscous
- Oats

Lean Proteins:

- Fatty fish (salmon, mackerel, sardines)
- Skinless poultry (chicken, turkey)
- Legumes (chickpeas, lentils, black beans)
- Tofu
- Eggs

Healthy Fats:

- Extra virgin olive oil
- Nuts (almonds, walnuts)
- Seeds (chia seeds, flaxseeds)
- Olives

Dairy and Dairy Alternatives:

- Greek yogurt
- Feta cheese
- Goat cheese
- Low-fat or plant-based milk

Herbs and Spices:

- Basil
- Oregano
- Mint
- Rosemary
- Thyme
- Cumin
- Paprika
- Turmeric

Sweeteners:

- Honey
- Maple syrup
- Dates

Fresh Herbs and Aromatics:

- Garlic
- Onion
- Parsley
- Dill
- Cilantro

Beverages:

- Red wine (moderate consumption)
- Herbal teas

<u>**Miscellaneous:**</u>

- Artichoke hearts (canned or frozen)
- Capers
- Sun-dried tomatoes
- Hummus
- Whole-grain pita bread

<u>Tips for a Successful Mediterranean Diet Grocery Shopping:</u>

Accept Colorful Produce: Pay close attention to a variety of vividly colored fruits and veggies. These form the basis of the Mediterranean diet and include a wide range of vitamins, minerals, and antioxidants.

Choose Whole Grains: Choose whole grains like farro, quinoa, and brown rice. These high-nutrient choices provide sustained energy and fullness.

Make Eating Lean Proteins Your Main Concern: Pick lean protein sources such as lentils, poultry, fatty fish, and tofu. These choices offer a well-rounded consumption of all the essential nutrients.

Select Healthy Fats: Essential items for your shopping basket should include nuts, seeds, and extra virgin olive oil. Sustaining heart health and overall well-being requires these heart-healthy lipids.

Look into Mediterranean Dairy: Put Greek yogurt, feta cheese, and goat cheese on your shopping list. These dairy products are a fantastic fit for the Mediterranean diet.

Invest in a Variety of Spices and Herbs: These additions may enhance the flavor of your cuisine. Herbs such as basil, oregano, mint, and others enhance flavor and offer nutritional benefits to food.

Conscious Sweeteners: Use natural sweeteners like dates, honey, and maple syrup sparingly. These sweet, well-balanced sweets complement a Mediterranean diet perfectly.

Use fresh herbs like parsley, onion, and garlic for making aromatics. Foods with these flavor-enhancing additives have intense flavors.

Add Mediterranean basics: Don't forget to include pantry basics like canned artichoke hearts, capers, and sun-dried tomatoes. These items add flavor and versatility to your meals.

Drink Herbal Teas to Stay Hydrated: Rich in antioxidants, herbal teas are a hydrating beverage option.

With this comprehensive shopping list, you'll be ready to fill your basket with the nutritious items that make up the Mediterranean diet. As you navigate the aisles, savor the thrill of cooking hearty, satisfying meals that fit within this traditional and healthy culinary lifestyle

2nd GIFT: 30-Day Quick Start Meal Plan for Weight Loss

Note: Feel free to change ingredients to fit your tastes and modify serving sizes to meet your specific requirements. This meal plan can be modified to fit specific dietary requirements or preferences; it is just intended to be a guide. It's also critical to stay hydrated throughout the day by drinking lots of water for weight loss and general wellness.

Day	Breakfast	Optional Snacks	Lunch	Dinner	Optional Dessert
1	Greek Yogurt Parfait	Handful of Almonds	Grilled Chicken Salad	Baked Salmon with Quinoa	Fresh Berries
2	Scrambled Eggs with Spinach	Apple Slices with Nut Butter	Quinoa and Black Bean Bowl	Mediterranean Vegetable Stir-Fry	Dark Chocolate-Dipped Strawberries
3	Oatmeal with Berries	Greek Yogurt with Honey	Lentil Soup with Whole Grain Bread	Grilled Turkey Breast with Roasted Vegetables	Orange Slices
4	Avocado Toast with Poached Egg	Cottage Cheese with Pineapple	Chickpea and Spinach Stew	Grilled Shrimp with Caulifl	Mixed Nuts

				ower Rice	
5	Whole Wheat Pancakes with Blueberries	Carrot Sticks with Hummus	Quinoa Salad with Feta Cheese	Mediterranean Baked Chicken	Frozen Yogurt with Fresh Mango
6	Smoothie Bowl with Spinach and Berries	Handful of Grapes	Greek Salad with Grilled Chicken	Zucchini Noodles with Tomato Sauce and Grilled Fish	Baked Apple Slices
7	Vegetable Omelette	Cherry Tomatoes with Mozzarella	Hummus and Veggie Wrap	Lentil and Vegetable Curry	Chia Seed Pudding with Mango
8	Whole Grain Cereal with Milk	Celery Sticks with Peanut Butter	Spinach and Quinoa Stuffed Bell Peppers	Baked Cod with Lemon and Herbs	Yogurt Parfait with Granola
9	Quinoa Breakfast Bowl	Banana with Almond Butter	Turkey and Avocado Wrap	Grilled Eggplant and Tomato	Fresh Mango Slices

				Stack	
10	Cottage Cheese and Pineapple	Greek Yogurt with Walnuts	Mediterranean Pasta Salad	Lemon Herb Chicken with Brown Rice	Berry Sorbet
11	Whole Wheat Toast with Avocado	Orange Slices	Tomato and Mozzarella Salad	Baked Zucchini Boats with Ground Turkey	Dark Chocolate Square
12	Scrambled Tofu with Vegetables	Handful of Almonds	Quinoa and Chickpea Buddha Bowl	Grilled Salmon with Asparagus	Greek Yogurt with Berries
13	Overnight Chia Seed Pudding	Carrot Sticks with Hummus	Greek Chicken Gyros	Mediterranean Stuffed Peppers	Baked Peach Halves
14	Almond Butter Banana Smoothie Bowl	Greek Yogurt with Honey	Lentil and Vegetable Soup	Baked Cod with Quinoa Pilaf	Mixed Berry Parfait
15	Whole Grain Waffles	Apple Slices with	Grilled Vegetable and	Chicken and Vegeta	Frozen Grapes

	with Berries	Almond Butter	Quinoa Bowl	ble Skewers	
16	Avocado and Tomato Toast	Cottage Cheese with Berries	Caprese Salad with Grilled Chicken	Spaghetti Squash with Tomato Sauce	Yogurt with Sliced Kiwi
17	Berry and Spinach Smoothie	Handful of Grapes	Hummus and Veggie Plate	Mediterranean Baked Fish	Dark Chocolate-Dipped Banana
18	Vegetable Frittata	Celery Sticks with Peanut Butter	Chickpea and Spinach Salad	Quinoa Stuffed Bell Peppers	Fresh Pineapple Chunks
19	Greek Yogurt Parfait	Orange Slices	Whole Wheat Wrap with Turkey and Avocado	Baked Chicken with Lemon and Herbs	Mango Sorbet
20	Scrambled Eggs with Spinach and Feta	Mixed Nuts	Quinoa Salad with Chickpeas	Grilled Shrimp and Vegetable Skewer	Yogurt with Berries

				s	
21	Oatmeal with Sliced Almonds	Greek Yogurt with Granola	Mediterranean Hummus Bowl	Baked Eggplant Parmesan	Dark Chocolate-Dipped Strawberries
22	Avocado and Berry Smoothie Bowl	Carrot Sticks with Hummus	Spinach and Feta Stuffed Chicken Breast	Grilled Salmon with Quinoa Salad	Fresh Mango Slices
23	Whole Wheat Pancakes with Blueberries	Apple Slices with Nut Butter	Lentil and Vegetable Curry	Mediterranean Grilled Vegetables	Baked Apple Slices
24	Smoothie Bowl with Spinach and Berries	Cottage Cheese with Pineapple	Greek Salad with Grilled Chicken	Baked Cod with Tomato and Olive Salsa	Frozen Yogurt with Fresh Berries
25	Vegetable Omelette	Cherry Tomatoes with Mozzarella	Quinoa and Black Bean Bowl	Grilled Turkey Breast with Roasted Vegetables	Orange Slices
26	Quinoa	Banana	Mediterra	Lemon	Chia

	Breakfast Bowl	with Almond Butter	nean Pasta Salad	Herb Chicken with Brown Rice	Seed Pudding with Mango
27	Cottage Cheese and Pineapple	Greek Yogurt with Walnuts	Hummus and Veggie Wrap	Lentil and Vegetable Soup	Mixed Nuts
28	Whole Wheat Toast with Avocado	Orange Slices	Tomato and Mozzarella Salad	Baked Zucchini Boats with Ground Turkey	Dark Chocolate Square
29	Scrambled Tofu with Vegetables	Handful of Almonds	Quinoa and Chickpea Buddha Bowl	Grilled Salmon with Asparagus	Greek Yogurt with Berries
30	Overnight Chia Seed Pudding	Carrot Sticks with Hummus	Greek Chicken Gyros	Mediterranean Stuffed Peppers	Baked Peach Halves

3rd GIF: Recipes Index